Lina Montaño
Julia Andrade
Gloria Roncallo

Biopsychosocial model as an interdisciplinary approach strategy

Lina Montaño
Julia Andrade
Gloria Roncallo

Biopsychosocial model as an interdisciplinary approach strategy

In orphan diseases

ScienciaScripts

Imprint
Any brand names and product names mentioned in this book are subject to trademark, brand or patent protection and are trademarks or registered trademarks of their respective holders. The use of brand names, product names, common names, trade names, product descriptions etc. even without a particular marking in this work is in no way to be construed to mean that such names may be regarded as unrestricted in respect of trademark and brand protection legislation and could thus be used by anyone.

Cover image: www.ingimage.com

This book is a translation from the original published under ISBN 978-613-9-46663-4.

Publisher:
Sciencia Scripts
is a trademark of
Dodo Books Indian Ocean Ltd. and OmniScriptum S.R.L publishing group

120 High Road, East Finchley, London, N2 9ED, United Kingdom
Str. Armeneasca 28/1, office 1, Chisinau MD-2012, Republic of Moldova, Europe
Printed at: see last page
ISBN: 978-620-8-33324-9

METROPOLITAN UNIVERSITY BARRANQUILLA/ATLANTICO

AUTHORS

Lina María Montaño Henao. Occupational Therapist, Specialist in school learning and its difficulties, Master in learning difficulties. Mail :lmontanoh@unimetro.edu.co, https://orcid.org/0000-0002-0097-5882 Affiliation: Universidad Metropolitana Country Colombia

Julia Andrade Orozco, Physiotherapist, Master in occupational health and safety, Mail: jandradeo@unimetro.edu.co, https://orcid.org/0000-0002-3847- 0554, Affiliation: Universidad Metropolitana Country Colombia

Gloria Roncallo Duran, Nutritionist and Dietitian, specialist in University Teaching and Master in Food and Nutrition Security groncallo@unimetro.edu.co, https://orcid.org/0000-003-3500-5279 Affiliation: Universidad Metropolitana Country Colombia

Margarita Rosa Larios Solórzano, Physiotherapist, Specialist in project management, Candidate for Master's degree in education, Contact e-mail: margarita.larios@unimetro.edu.co, https://orcid.org/0000-0003-2860-7018 Affiliation: Universidad Metropolitana Country Colombia

Yesenia Milena Manotas Guzmán, Speech therapist, Master in disability, Master in inclusive and intercultural education, Specialist in educational games and hearing rehabilitation, Mail: yessenia.manotas@unimetro.edu.co, Orcid https://orcid.org/0000-0002-0576-0936 Affiliation: Universidad Metropolitana Country Colombia

Karen Bolaño Diaz, Social Worker, Specialist in university teaching, Candidate for a Master's degree in education. Mail: kbolano@unimetro.edu.co, Orcid https://orcid.org/0009-0005-9587-3297 Affiliation: Universidad Metropolitana Country Colombia

Miguel Alberto Montañez Romero, Psychologist, Master in Psychoneuropsychiatry and Rehabilitation, PhD Candidate in Applied Cognitive Neurosciences miguel.montanez@unimetro.edu.co, Mail: miguel.montanez@unimetro.edu.co, Orcid https://orcid.org/0000-0002-4534-4515 Affiliation: Universidad Metropolitana Country Colombia

SUMMARY

Orphan diseases, also known as rare diseases, are medical conditions that are usually chronic, debilitating and, in many cases, lack specific treatments due to their low prevalence, affecting a very limited number of people compared to the general population. The aim of this study was to analyze which rehabilitation processes, intervention and biopsychosocial models have the greatest applicability in people suffering from orphan diseases. This will be done through a methodology based on a documentary review of qualitative-descriptive typology. The PRISMA method was used for the collection of systematic reviews. Among the results, it was possible to recognize the different affectations of orphan diseases, allowing the interprofessional approach and the benefits in care and rehabilitation, to improve the quality of life of patients. As conclusions, the information gathered becomes a valuable resource for health professionals, researchers and those involved in decision making related to medical care in rare diseases. By thoroughly understanding the complexities of these diseases, it paves the way for the creation of more effective and personalized treatment protocols, thus improving the quality of life for those facing these challenging medical conditions.

Keywords: Rare Diseases; Orphan Diseases; Rehabilitation; Disability; Intervention; Biopsychosocial Model.

Table of Contents

INTRODUCTION

Rare or orphan diseases are those that are detected in every 5 out of 10,000 people (Mejía et al., 2018). One of their characteristics is that they appear at an early age, due to diseases of genetic origin and congenital anomalies, however, it is necessary to mention that the prevalence of these is higher in adults than in children, due to the high mortality rate of some of these diseases in children and the influence of certain diseases, which arise at late ages. Viteri, et.al (2020), recognize that these diseases have been throughout history, however, at the end of the 20th century, these genetic diseases and those that present genetic components have emerged as a significant cause of morbidity and mortality in the western world. According to the author, this change in the health landscape has led to a greater understanding of the complexity of conditions linked to genetics, marking a transition towards identifying and addressing diseases that have their roots in the genetic material of individuals.

However, it is essential to note that the notion of "rare" diseases was first introduced in the United States in the mid-1980s. This term was simultaneously associated with the notion of "orphan" drugs, pointing to the scarce research and production around these diseases (Hermoso, 2021). This lack of attention has resulted in those suffering from these pathologies experiencing considerable difficulties in resolving their health problems.

Within this context, it is estimated that around 4,000 of these diseases lack a curative treatment. (Hermoso, 2021) This situation is a substantial challenge in the medical field, as the lack of therapeutic options leaves affected patients and their families vulnerable, often dealing with health conditions for which medical science has not yet found conclusive answers. (Posada, et. al 2008). Thus, the concept of rare diseases is not only linked to the rarity of their incidence, but also to the limitations in research and development of treatments to effectively address these rare medical conditions (Carrasco & Fernanda, 2020).

Orphan diseases, for the most part, are characterized by being chronic and progressive (Hermoso, 2021; Posada, 2008; Viteri et al., 2020), with some of them presenting significant early mortality rates (Viteri et al., 2020), while others can generate severe motor, sensory and cognitive disabilities (Antonia & Nadal, 2018) even in a short period. The diversity of these diseases, together with their clinical complexity and low frequency in the population, poses substantial challenges in several aspects.

In addition, limited access to diagnostic tests and treatments represents another crucial obstacle. In many cases, the availability of specific medical resources for these diseases is scarce, which further complicates early identification and appropriate management, in addition, the lack of sufficient scientific information available on these rare diseases contributes to uncertainty regarding their underlying mechanisms and effective treatment options (Hirmas et al., 2013).

These challenges not only affect patients, but also place significant pressure on healthcare systems, as the need for specialized and high-cost care to address these rare diseases places a considerable economic burden on healthcare systems, which must adapt to provide specific services and necessary resources (Hirmas et al., 2013). This scenario is compounded by the emotional and social implications that these diseases entail for patients and their families, who often face a lack of support and understanding in society, as well as additional financial challenges associated with the costs of treatment and long-term care.

Recognizing their incidence in only 6-8% of the world's population, rare diseases present a number of characteristics that distinguish them in a remarkable way, contributing to their complexity from both a medical and social perspective (Castañeda, 2023). Beyond their low prevalence in numerical terms, these conditions are characterized by significant challenges that affect the lives of those who suffer from them (Castañeda, 2023).

Diagnostic difficulty arises as a first distinctive element (Tejada-Ortigosa et al., 2019). The rarity of their manifestations and generalized knowledge about these conditions complicate their identification and contribute to delays in diagnosis, negatively affecting the timely implementation of appropriate treatments (Tejada-Ortigosa et al., 2019). Likewise, the limited availability of therapeutic alternatives emerges as a second distinctive feature, since they lack specific treatments, which not only impacts the quality of life of patients, but also increases the economic burden associated with specialized and costly treatments that are often necessary (Tejada-Ortigosa et al., 2019).

In addition, these conditions tend to be severe, chronic and progressive, presenting ongoing health challenges for those affected. Manifestations may be present from birth or infancy, but they can also emerge in adulthood, adding an additional layer of complexity to their identification and management. It is crucial to note that most rare diseases have a genetic component, although the influence of the environment on their development cannot be ruled out. This interaction between genetic and environmental factors adds a dimension of complexity to these conditions, which are unique in their variety.

A significant challenge facing those living with rare diseases is the widespread lack of information and knowledge about their conditions (Viteri et al., 2020). This gap manifests itself even at the primary levels of medical care, further complicating the diagnostic process and exacerbating the uncertainty surrounding these diseases. The study of these diseases contributes significantly to gaining an understanding of their characteristics for intervention.

Approaching the analysis of orphan diseases from a rehabilitation and intervention perspective based on the biopsychosocial model is of fundamental importance in the comprehensive care of affected patients. In other words, the aim of this review is to analyze the processes of rehabilitation and intervention under the biopsychosocial model. First, the rehabilitation processes of patients and their improvement of quality of life are analyzed, and then the methods of intervention, which include both clinical and non-clinical, the specific needs of each person. Also, the factors that allow a deeper understanding of these diseases are analyzed, in order to facilitate strategies for the patient's development.

For this reason, it is necessary to review the different biopsychosocial implications that may affect rehabilitation processes, since rehabilitation is an essential component to improve the quality of life of patients, since it seeks to maximize their functionality and autonomy despite the limitations imposed by the disease. Intervention, on the other hand, focuses on providing treatments and support tailored to the specific needs of each individual, considering both physical and emotional aspects. The biopsychosocial model allows a more complete understanding of rare diseases, facilitating more comprehensive and patient-centered treatment strategies, including rehabilitation, promoting their integration into society.

METHODOLOGY

For the development of this research, a qualitative-descriptive methodology has been established (Sampieri et al., 2004). This methodology is presented as an essential tool in the analysis of rehabilitation processes, intervention and psychosocial models associated with orphan diseases. It allows capturing the complexities and nuances of patients' experiences, as well as the social dynamics that influence their adaptation (Sampieri et al., 2004).

This research approach allows a deep and contextualized understanding of the information gathered (Sampieri et al., 2004) from case studies, indexed information on orphan diseases, as well as the various factors that influence their rehabilitation process and the effectiveness of interventions.

In the context of orphan diseases, where case diversity and paucity of information are notable (Llanos et al, 2020), this methodology becomes critical to identify patterns, challenges and key issues that can meaningfully inform rehabilitation and intervention approaches.

On the other hand, in the process of obtaining information on rehabilitation, intervention and biopsychosocial models in the context of orphan diseases, an exhaustive documentary review will be carried out, with relevant data from various sources, including studies, reports and specialized documents, exploration of scientific journals and the use of meta-search engines specialized in medical information. The databases used for the collection of information are PubMed, Scopus, Web of Science, ScienceDirect, among others.

Likewise, it is crucial to highlight that the temporal focus will be limited to the last five years, ensuring the inclusion of recent research and advances in the field of orphan diseases. In addition, the search for information will be conducted in multiple languages, such as Spanish and English, with the aim of covering a wider range of knowledge and perspectives on the topic (Álvarez- Hernández et al., 2021).

It is important to note that the most recurrent terms for the collection of information cover a wide range of diseases, focusing particularly on those related to the nervous system, disorders of the blood and hematopoietic organs, congenital malformations, deformities and chromosomal anomalies, endocrine, nutritional and metabolic diseases, as well as those related to the musculoskeletal system and connective tissue.

The breadth of terms used reflects the diversity of rare diseases and, at the same time, the need for a thorough understanding of the different medical and biopsychosocial aspects associated with them. In addition, emphasis is placed on the importance of exploring not only the diseases themselves, but also the type of intervention applied, as well as the biopsychosocial adaptation models that have been developed in the field of rehabilitation. This comprehensive approach allows the complexities of orphan diseases to be addressed from different perspectives, including both clinical aspects and those related to quality of life, psychological adaptation and intervention strategies. The diversity of terms and the inclusion of diverse fields reflect a commitment to a comprehensive and accurate view that enriches the understanding of these rare medical conditions.

In methodological terms, the search is guided by the PRISMA method, following the updated version of the year 2020 (Farrús, 2023). The PRISMA method (Preferred Reporting Items for Systematic Reviews and Meta-Analyses) establishes rigorous guidelines for conducting systematic reviews, ensuring a transparent and reproducible process (Farrús, 2023). This methodology seeks not only to compile high-quality information, but also to provide an accurate and complete synthesis of the most current advances in the field of rehabilitation, intervention and biopsychosocial models related to orphan diseases (Álvarez-Hernández et al., 2021; Farrús, 2023). Likewise, for the structuring of the information, the Excel office automation tool is used, which systematically organizes and structures the information collected. The structure selected for this article is the name(s) of the author(s), year of publication, title of the research, objective, methodology and results.

In the process of selecting information for the review, the importance of the inclusion and exclusion criteria that guide the identification and collection of relevant data is emphasized (Sampieri et al., 2004). In terms of inclusion, priority is given to documentary and scientific information available in Spanish and English, with the aim of covering a variety of perspectives and studies in different languages in the medical field. The search focuses on publications in indexed journals, ensuring the quality and validity of the information collected, as well as publications on Internet pages of recognized media in the medical sector, thus providing a broader and updated perspective on the topics of interest (Álvarez-Hernández et al., 2021; Sampieri et al., 2004).

It is important to highlight that the information search process for this study was based on the selection of relevant keywords that would allow a comprehensive approach to the topic of rare diseases and rehabilitation, especially from the perspective of the biopsychosocial model of intervention.

The keyword combinations selected for the Spanish research were the following: "Enfermedades raras" AND "rehabilitación", "Avances", "Modelo biopsicosocial", "intervención.", "Integrando el modelo biopsicosocial en enfermedades huérfanas y rehabilitación.", "Rehabilitación" AND "enfermedades raras: Perspectivas desde el modelo biopsicosocial.", "Enfermedades huérfanas", "rehabilitación" AND "enfoque de intervención biopsicosocial.", and "Modelo biopsicosocial" AND "rehabilitación", "enfermedades raras.", and "Modelo biopsicosocial" AND "rehabilitación", "enfermedades raras". Each of these combinations was designed to capture specific and relevant aspects of the topic, thus allowing for a comprehensive and detailed exploration; and to include international perspectives and enrich the analysis with research and scientific approaches from diverse sources, "Integrating the biopsychosocial model in orphan diseases AND rehabilitation.", "Rehabilitation AND rare diseases: Perspectives from the biopsychosocial model.", "Orphan diseases, rehabilitation, AND the biopsychosocial intervention approach.", AND "Exploring the biopsychosocial model in the rehabilitation of rare diseases.", AND "Exploring the biopsychosocial model in the rehabilitation of rare diseases.".

In the initial phase of this research process, a review of the scientific literature was conducted, where 50 articles related to rare diseases and rehabilitation were selected. This initial approach was essential to cover a wide range of studies and perspectives in the field. However, upon careful analysis, it was identified that, among the 50 initial articles, only 20 stood out for their significant relevance, substantial findings and pertinent contributions to the conceptual framework of the research.

These 20 articles, which emerged as essential for the construction of knowledge, have been detailed and presented in an organized manner in Table 1.

Table 1. Search results

Author's name	Year of publication	Title of research	Target	Methodology	Results
Mamala dze Mamala dze, T	2022	Neuropsychological assessment and rehabilitation in multiple sclerosis	Minimize emotional, behavioral and cognitive difficulties to minimize the impact on the daily life of people with multiple sclerosis, improving their family, work and social environment.	The methodology used in this study is based on an exhaustive evaluation of the patient, using neuropsychological assessment tools and techniques. A detailed description of the pathology, Multiple Sclerosis, is presented and the most relevant results obtained during the evaluation are discussed. The proposed intervention includes 48 sessions over 6 months, each lasting approximately 40 minutes.	The neuropsychological evaluation reveals that the patient has marked difficulties in several cognitive areas, such as attention, concentration and speed of information processing. Alterations in executive functions and memory are observed, as well as marked fatigue. These results support the need for a specific neuropsychological intervention (Mamaladz et al., 2022). The intervention plan has been designed with the aim of reducing these emotional, behavioral and cognitive difficulties, as well as minimizing the impact on the patient's daily life. The proposed cognitive rehabilitation strategy will be implemented over six months, seeking not only to optimize the patient's preserved skills, but also to improve her quality of life and promote her autonomy in different contexts (Mamaladz et al.,

					2022).
Pérez Cerdán , G.	2023	Visual rehabilitation for people with Multiple Sclerosis	bibliographic review to know the efficiency of rehabilitation in patients with Multiple Scleriosis.	Systematic review of 16 articles.	In the rehabilitation process of patients with Multiple Sclerosis (MS), a number of significant benefits have been observed. In particular, the incorporation of video games in the intervention has been shown to improve the cognitive and psychological function of MS patients, showing a similar effectiveness to that observed in the control group. The results indicate notable improvements in motor function, with small differences in gait speed and stride time after the application of virtual rehabilitation therapy (Master's Degree in Visual Rehabilitation, n.d.). Accuracy and consistency experienced noticeable improvements, especially under conditions 19 combined (Master's Degree in Visual Rehabilitation, n.d.). In addition, an improvement in sensory and motor information processing has been reported,

					highlighting a positive impact on motor and cognitive skills. Patients reported a reduction in diplopia and an improvement in quality of life, thus indicating the therapeutic and motivational value of this rehabilitation modality in the context of Multiple Sclerosis (Master's Degree in Visual Rehabilitation, n.d.).
Acosta Plasce nc ia, K. M.	2021	Effects of neuropsychological rehabilitation on a patient with multiple sclerosis	case analysis of neuropsychological rehabilitation in a patient with multiple sclerosis	Assessments were performed both before and after the intervention to obtain a complete perspective of the effects of the program. In the first assessment, the patient's primary defect, related to regulation and control mechanisms, and secondary impairments in audio-verbal and visual retention analyzers, as well as in intellectual activity, were identified.	At the neuropsychological level, significant improvements were highlighted in the primary factor of regulation and control, as well as in the audio-verbal retention factors **(20210416160 802-2566-T, s/f).** At the psychological level, the analysis of the patient's primary defect, related to the regulation and control mechanisms, and the secondary affectations in the audio-verbal and visual retention analyzers, as well as in the intellectual activity structure of the activity revealed a positive effect in each link, from orientation to verification. These findings indicate that the intervention had a

					positive impact on both cognitive and psychological levels **(*2021041 6160802-2566-T, s/***, highlighting the effectiveness of the program in improving the mechanisms of regulation and control, as well as in the quality of the patient's intellectual activity as a result of the intervention. **EM(*2021041616082-2566-T, s/f*).**
Farioli, M. E., & Rueda, U. A.	2023	Effects of kinesic rehabilitation on musculoskeletal aspects in adult patients with hemophilia.	To conduct a comprehensive review of the existing literature on the impacts of various kinesthetic interventions used in the management of musculoskeletal problems in individuals affected by hemophilia.	The search strategy was carried out in the recognized databases of PubMed, the Virtual Health Library (VHL) and the SciELO system. The selection of articles was limited to those available in full text, published between 2010 and 2022, and written in English or Spanish. After an exhaustive review and selection process, nine articles were identified and considered for analysis.	significant improvement in joint pain management was evidenced. In addition, improvements in range of motion (ROM) were observed, indicating benefits in mobility and flexibility. articulate **(*Inv. D-398 MFN 7614 tesis, s/*** Likewise, the frequency of joint bleeding (hemarthrosis) was favored. These findings underline the importance and potential efficacy of kinesthetic interventions in the management of musculoskeletal conditions in patients with hemophilia, providing key perspectives for the improvement of

					treatment and quality of life of these individuals (Inv. **D-398 MFN 76 tesis, s/f).**
Gonzál e z Coquel , S., Fortich Gonzál e z, R., Castill o Garrid o, B., Laurie, J. C., Pinzón Consue g ra, J., Aparici o Maren co , D. E., & Díaz Beltrán , G. R.	2023	Orphan-rare diseases, physiopathology and complications of some that compromise the health and quality of life and the processes for the care of infants who suffer from them.	examine the situation of people affected by Orphan Diseases (OD).	The methodology used in this research is descriptive and based on a quantitative approach. Information was collected through an exhaustive review of the scientific literature, using databases such as PubMed and the Virtual Health Library (VHL). Data from the World Health Organization (WHO) and Latin American collaborative studies on congenital malformations were considered to provide a comprehensive view of the HD situation.	Research reveals that HD affects approximately 7% of the world's population, representing about 500 million people(REGISTRAT ION FORM DOCUMENT CONSOLIDATED PAT COLLECTIVE, n/d). In Latin America, these diseases are among the main causes of mortality in children under 1 year of age. Worldwide, between 6000 and 8000 orphan diseases have been identified, and 2198 pathologies have been registered in Colombia(FORMAT O REGISTRO DOCUMENT CONSOLIDATED PAT COLLECTIVE, n/d). The lack of cures and palliative treatments, coupled with the high cost of treatments not covered by the national health system, places patients in conditions of social and institutional neglect. The research highlights the urgency of

					overcoming the barriers to access to health services for these patients, underlining the importance of addressing the neglect and institutional abandonment faced by people with HD(FORMAT REGISTRY DOCUMENT CONSOLIDATED PAT COLLECTIVE, n/d).
Lagunas, M. C.	2022	Nursing care process executed in a patient with Guillain-Barré Syndrome admitted to an intensive care unit.	to understand the specific and potential needs of a man in the critical phase of Guillain-Barré syndrome while admitted to an intensive care unit (ICU).	bibliographic review in the main scientific databases, focusing on Guillain-Barré syndrome and intensive care unit (ICU). nursing care for patients admitted to intensive care units (ICU). The information collected was limited to the last 10 years to ensure the relevance and timeliness of the data.	he nursing care provided to the patient with Guillain-Barré syndrome during his stay in the intensive care unit (ICU) focused on the comprehensive management of both clinical and psychological signs and symptoms (Final Degree Project, n.d.). This approach not only focused on the patient, but also actively involved the family in the therapeutic process (Final Degree Project, n/d). Multidisciplinary collaboration, especially led by the nursing team, was crucial to minimize the complications and sequelae associated with the syndrome, thus improving the

					patient's quality of life during the hospital stay (Final Degree Project, n/d).
Camelo, L. R., Carpio, M. T., Camelo, L. R., & Carpio, M. T.	2023	Systematic Review of the Effectiveness of Physiotherapeutic Intervention through Telerehabilitation in Users with Neuromuscular System Impairment	To analyze the efficacy of physical therapy using telerehabilitation in individuals with neuromuscular system problems, using a systematic review approach.	Quantitative systematic review. The population addressed in this review is determined from the various results found in the selected research sources, while the sample is composed of original scientific articles derived from these investigations.	It is observed that performing exercises at home contributes significantly to strengthening muscles, improving range of motion and making progress in motor skills. The active participation of patients and their families stands out as a crucial factor in this process (Ramos Camelo María Taborda Carpio, n/d).
Flores, N. Y. S.	2021	Comprehensive neuropsychological rehabilitation in middle-aged adults with ischemic cerebrovascular disease.	To create and implement a comprehensive neuropsychological rehabilitation program with the aim of reducing or halting the cognitive consequences of ischemic cerebrovascular disease in middle-aged adults.	comprehensive neuropsychological rehabilitation program aimed at reducing or halting the cognitive consequences of ischemic cerebrovascular disease in middle-aged adults. This study adopts a quantitative and prospective pre-experimental and therapeutic approach. It was carried out by measuring a single group at two different	significant improvements were observed in orientation, language, mental calculation, verbal memory, executive functions and processing speed. Although attention did not show statistically significant changes, it was preserved at the clinical level. In addition, depressive symptomatology decreased, reaching mild levels, and anxiety states, initially prominent, showed functional and clinical improvement,

				times: before and after the intervention.	especially in cases of moderate depression at the beginning (Yetlanezi Salazar Flores et al., n/d).
Carro Castiñe ir a, T.	2021	Impact of biopsychosocial factors on the quality of life of people diagnosed with fibromyalgia.	to analyze the impact of biopsychosocial factors on the quality of life (QoL) of individuals diagnosed with fibromyalgia (FM).	A qualitative methodology based on the phenomenologic al approach was used. The study was carried out at the AFFINOR association, Using ad hoc surveys administered to selected users. The results obtained were analyzed using the Atlas.TI program.	The participants revealed significant limitations in occupational areas such as instrumental activities of daily living, work, rest and sleep, leisure, free time and social participation (Vila Paz et al., n/d). Sexual activity was identified as particularly affected in this group. Variables such as "cognitive impairment", "degree of support" and "economic situation" showed a direct relationship with self-perceived symptoms, QOL and occupational performance (Vila Paz et al., n/d).
Velard e García, M.	2023	Nursing care in neonates with bronchopulmona ry dysplasia in an Essalud hospital.	to determine the relationship between nursing care provided to neonates diagnosed with bronchopulmona ry dysplasia at the EsSalud Lima hospital during the year 2022.	descriptive methodology that focuses on describing the relationship between the selected variables. The research will follow a general inductive-deductive method, combined with	It is essential to provide adequate nursing care to preterm infants, as this plays a key role in reducing the impact and possible sequelae of bronchopulmonary dysplasia on their future development (UNIVERSID AD INCA GARCILASO DE LA VEGA, n/d).

				the use of statistical methods to facilitate the representation of observed data. A non-experimental, transectional, descriptive and correlational design will be used. Population.	Bronchopulmonary dysplasia, a disease that specifically affects premature infants, highlights the crucial importance of prevention and timely treatment, especially through specialized and individualized care (UNI VERSIDAD INCA GARCILASO DE LA VEGA, n.d.).
Díaz Chamba, W. I., & Mena Noroña, D. A.	2023	Demographic and clinical characteristics and management of pediatric patients with a diagnosis of microtia seen at the Otorhinolaryngology Department of the Baca Ortiz Pediatric Hospital.	To analyze the demographic and clinical characteristics and the management of pediatric patients with a diagnosis of microtia seen at the Otorhinolaryngology Department of the Baca Ortiz Pediatric Hospital.	Observational and descriptive cross-sectional study with analysis of qualitative variables. The study population included pediatric patients with a diagnosis of microtia seen in the Otorhinolaryngology area of the Baca Ortiz Pediatric Hospital.	the preferential involvement of the right pinna (57%) stood out (Demográficas et al., n/d). The presence of hypoacusis was significant, manifesting in 99.1% of the cases. In addition, a statistically significant association was identified between geographic altitude and the presence of microtia, with the highlands region of Ecuador concentrating 94% of the cases, Quito being the most affected city with 53.2% (Demográficas et al., n/d).
Buono, M. P.	2020	Physiotherapy treatments in Focal Dystonia of the musician's hand.	to review the available scientific evidence on physiotherapeuti	literature review in various databases, including PUBMED, ,	a wide variety of physiotherapeutic treatments have been identified for Focal Hand Dystonia in

		Bibliographic review.	c treatments for Focal Hand Dystonia in musicians, with the aim of identifying the most effective combination of such treatments.	DIALNET, ENFISPO and COCHRANE LIBRARY. The review period spanned from 2015 to the current date.	musicians, none of which have strong evidence of effectiveness (-------- ------------------------ -). ------------------------ - ------------------------ - ------------------------ - ------- et al., n/d). Treatments that incorporate the combination of several techniques and/or methods appear to be more effective than those that apply one technique in isolation (--------------- -------- -----------------). ------------------------ - ------------------------ - ------------------------ et al., n.d.).
Peron-Magna n, T.	2023	Rehabilitation of dystonia.	address dystonias, which are part of the abnormal involuntary movements, exploring their various manifestations, etiologies and treatments of Dystonia.	The study is descriptive and analytical, focusing on dystonias and their phenotypes according to the current international classification. The main circumstances surrounding the dystonias are reviewed and specific rehabilitation approaches are	The application of muscle stretching and strengthening techniques has been shown to be beneficial in improving dystonia symptoms in musicians. These specific exercises focus on the affected musculature, seeking to improve muscle flexibility and strength(Huasasquic he et al., 2017)r. In the context of focal hand dystonia in

				explored, with a particular emphasis on cervical dystonia and writer's cramp. The methodology encompasses clinical analysis, rehabilitation techniques, the therapeutic relationship and interdisciplinary collaboration as key components.	musicians, regular implementation of stretching and strengthening routines has shown promising results by contributing to increased motor coordination and alleviating involuntary muscle contractions. This therapeutic approach not only aims to reduce symptoms, but also to improve functionality and performance in musical activities, providing musicians with a higher quality of life and well-being in their artistic practice(Huasasquic h e et al., 2017).
Neivis, T. H., Marian n e, S. S., & Ada, M. F.	2021	Dystonia and occupational therapeutic care.	analyze and understand the relationship between the prevalence of neuromuscular diseases and the socioeconomic conditions in a specific population	comprehensive review of epidemiological data, as well as analysis of relevant socioeconomic indicators. A representative sampling of the population will be carried out, gathering demographic and economic information that will allow meaningful connections to be established.	The results obtained so far indicate a significant correlation between unfavorable socioeconomic conditions and the prevalence of neuromuscular diseases in the population studied. It is observed that those sectors with limited resources face a higher risk of developing this type of disease (Torrie nte Herrera et al., n.d.).
Toro Ruiz,	2021	Evaluation and neuropsychologi	present the case of a 60-year-old	exhaustive neuropsychologi	The neuropsychological

C. D.		cal intervention in a case of corticobasal degeneration.	female patient with corticobasal degeneration (CBD) that has been evolving for 5 years.	cal evaluation of the patient, addressing cognitive, motor and emotional aspects. Based on the results obtained, a neuropsychological rehabilitation program consisting of 24 sessions distributed over 12 weeks is proposed.	evaluation revealed moderate/severe cognitive impairment, with predominant impairment in executive functions, learning and memory, praxias, visuospatial and visuoperceptive skills, as well as academic skills (Del Toro et al., 2021a). At the motor level, a wide range of symptoms was observed, including tremor, dystonia, myoclonus, rigidity, hypokinesia, spasticity and bradykinesia. Emotional assessment indicated elevated levels of depression and anxiety, along with moderate apathy (Del Toro et al., 2021a).
Domski Chiriboga, A. M.	2020	Community nutrition, life cycle, Crohn's disease and Down syndrome case development.	apply and consolidate the knowledge acquired throughout the nutrition career.	nutrition integration workshop involves the application of knowledge in four case studies, each focused on specific areas of nutrition. These cases cover a variety of settings, including community, public health, adult and pediatric	the acquired knowledge was effectively applied, providing a clearer vision on the practical application of nutrition in different scenarios **(María & Chiriboga, s/f)**. The cases presented allowed addressing relevant topics, such as the relationship between nutrition and pathophysiology, nutritional assessment in

				hospital settings, and private practice situations.	different contexts and counseling children, and private consultation situations. nutritionally adapted to the specific needs of each case **(María & Chiriboga, s/f).**
Hayduk, V. A., and Quintana , A.	2019	The professional intervention of Social Work in the rehabilitation process of people with Amyotrophic Lateral Sclerosis.	to describe the intervention of Social Work in the rehabilitation process of people with Amyotrophic Lateral Sclerosis (ALS). The importance of addressing this topic is highlighted, given the scarcity of exploration in the field of Social Work.	The methodology used in the article focuses on the detailed description of Social Work interventions with patients diagnosed with ALS. Patient experience stories, such as Juan's case, are included to illustrate how the disease affects daily life and independence. In addition, the importance of accompaniment and care by social workers is highlighted.	The results of the research highlight the importance of accompaniment, interdiscipline and constant training of the health care team in the intervention of social workers with patients diagnosed with ELA(*Hayduk-94, s/* It emphasizes the need for comprehensive health policies on the part of the State to improve the quality of life and social inclusion of people with disabilities. ELA(*Hayduk-94, s/*
de Armas, Á. U. L., Acosta, M. N., & Moinelo, M. C.	2021	Intervention strategy for memory rehabilitation in adults with amyotrophic lateral sclerosis.	to analyze the impact of rehabilitation strategies in patients with spinal cord injury.	qualitative approach, conducting in-depth interviews with individuals who have participated in rehabilitation programs, as well as with health professionals	Rehabilitation strategies discussed include physical, occupational and speech therapy, as well as psychological and social support programs (brief initial and final Mini-Mental State by the Department of Neuropsychology,

				specialized in spinal cord injury. In addition, a quantitative analysis of the data collected is carried out to identify patterns and trends in the effectiveness of different rehabilitation strategies.	n.d.). The effectiveness of these strategies in improving mobility, functional independence and quality of life of patients with spinal cord injury is evaluated (brief initial and final Mini-Mental State by the Department of Neuropsychology, n.d.).
Shigua n go Reyes, E. S.	2021	Respiratory physiotherapy in patients with Duchenne Muscular Dystrophy.	to analyze the efficacy of respiratory physiotherapy in patients with Duchenne muscular dystrophy (DMD).	exhaustive search of information in various scientific databases, including Science Direct ELSEVIER, ProQuest, WorldWideSci ence, Dianet, Google Scholar and PubMed. A total of 122 scientific articles were collected and subjected to a detailed analysis.	After the analysis of the information collected, it was concluded that physical therapy, especially the respiratory branch, is effective in the application to patients with Duchenne Muscular Dystrophy (DMD)(Yartú Couceiro, n/d). This practice is revealed as a valuable resource to improve the quality of life of patients by delaying the progression of the disease and promoting greater functionality in daily activities (Yartú Couceiro, n/d). Physiotherapy, through exercises and breathing techniques, is essential to improve pulmonary functionality, since the cardiorespiratory

					system is affected over time.

Source: own elaboration.

Each offers a valuable and specific contribution to understanding the interrelationships between rare diseases and rehabilitation, integrating the biopsychosocial model of intervention. This careful selection not only ensures the quality of the information collected, but also allows a precise focus on the most relevant and significant aspects of the study topic.

Nevertheless, to ensure the comprehensiveness and validity of the review, we recognize the importance of considering all of the 50 articles initially selected. Although some did not achieve the same prominence in terms of direct relevance, each investigation provided valuable perspectives and complementary data that enriched the overall understanding of the phenomenon studied. This strategy of taking advantage of the diversity of the scientific literature allows not only to solidly support the conclusions, but also to offer a comprehensive and contextualized view of the interactions between rare diseases and rehabilitation.

On the other hand, exclusion criteria are established to maintain the integrity and reliability of the information collected (Sampieri, 2004), since unverified information is excluded, guaranteeing the reliability of the data included in the review. Likewise, information published in non-scientific documents is disregarded, in order to maintain a rigorous approach based on scientific evidence. Web pages not recognized by medical institutions are discarded. These inclusion and exclusion criteria are meticulously applied to ensure the quality and relevance of the information collected in the review process.

RESULTS

Neuropsychological intervention

Neuropsychological rehabilitation in multiple sclerosis (MS) involves comprehensive processes that seek to address the cognitive and functional challenges associated with this disease (Mamaladze, 2022). In the medical setting, intervention focuses on strategies to mitigate cognitive symptoms, such as problems with memory, attention, and information processing (Mamaladze, 2022). Specific techniques and therapies led by health professionals, such as neuropsychologists and physiotherapists, are employed with the aim of optimizing brain function and improving the quality of life of MS patients.

At the family and social level, neuropsychological rehabilitation is not limited to the affected individual (Mamaladze, 2022), but involves his or her support network. Families play a crucial role in providing an emotionally and practically supportive environment, as family members' understanding of cognitive challenges enables the implementation of adaptive strategies in daily life. Family involvement in the rehabilitation process contributes to creating an environment conducive to the patient's well-being (Pizarro, 2013), furthermore, the importance of social intervention in the neuropsychological rehabilitation process in MS is highlighted (Pizarro, 2013). Community support programs, support groups and social services contribute to the integration and participation of affected individuals in society (Pizarro, 2013). Awareness and understanding of multiple sclerosis play a significant role in creating an inclusive and supportive environment for those living with this disease.

Within the context of neuropsychological rehabilitation in multiple sclerosis (MS), it has been observed that video games are presented as an innovative and effective tool to improve both cognitive and motor functions (Bove et al., 2019; Kalb et al., 2020; Menascu et al., 2021; Pallavicini et al., 2018), as well as motor and sensory information processing. These adaptive games can be specifically designed to address particular challenges associated with MS, providing an interactive platform that encompasses cognitive and motor aspects in a comprehensive manner (Bove et al., 2019).

From a cognitive perspective, video games can be targeted to areas such as memory, attention and information processing, providing gradual and adaptive challenges (Kalb et al., 2020; Menascu et al., 2021). This approach seeks to stimulate cognitive abilities affected by the disease, such as fostering brain plasticity and facilitating adaptation to neurodegenerative changes (Pallavicini et al., 2018). Regarding the motor domain, video games can be used with the aim of improving coordination, balance and dexterity, counteracting the effects of motor dysfunction linked to MS (Forsyth et al., 2020; Pallavicini et al., 2018; Scaturro et al., 2021). The interactivity of video games provides opportunities for controlled and repetitive practice of specific movements, which may be beneficial in maintaining or improving motor function.

In cases of diplopia, the incorporation of specifically designed video games can help reduce this symptom, since the adaptive visual exercises present in the games contribute to the improvement of vision and ocular coordination, generating a positive impact on quality of life by mitigating the effects of diplopia (Fernandez & Arcos, 2019; Pallavicini et al., 2018).

Within the framework of neuropsychological rehabilitation in MS (Fernandez & Arcos, 2019) it is crucial to highlight that, significant improvements in the control and retention of audio-verbal information have been observed as a result of therapeutic interventions, including the use of adaptive video games (Fernandez & Arcos, 2019). These games not only offer visual stimuli, but can also incorporate auditory elements (Pallavicini et al., 2018), providing a comprehensive platform to address specific challenges associated with MS.

In the field of social development, neuropsychological rehabilitation is not only limited to cognitive and motor aspects (Fernandez & Arcos, 2019), but also has a positive impact on orientation and information verification in the social environment (Rodriguez, B. 2019; Vila Paz et al., 2021). Participation in activities based on adaptive video games can facilitate social interaction, improve communication skills and promote teamwork, thus contributing to a more complete development at the cognitive and social level of individuals affected by MS. This integration of audiovisual elements in rehabilitation interventions not only diversifies therapeutic experiences, but also specifically adapts to the individual needs and challenges of each patient with multiple sclerosis (Fernandez & Arcos, 2019).

Physiotherapeutic Intervention

In the context of comprehensive treatment for patients with hemophilia, kinesthetic intervention emerges as an essential component, providing substantial benefits from both medical and biopsychosocial perspectives (Deniz et al., 2022; López-Casaus et al., 2021). From the medical field, kinesic rehabilitation contributes significantly to the management of joint pain in patients with hemophilia. Through adapted therapeutic programs, it focuses on strengthening the surrounding muscles and improving joint mobility, thus reducing the load and pressure on joints affected by recurrent bleeding. The application of specific physiotherapy techniques, such as strengthening and stretching exercises, helps to minimize pain intensity and optimize joint functionality (Del Toro et al., 2021).

From a biopsychosocial perspective, kinesic rehabilitation has a comprehensive impact on the lives of hemophilia patients. At the biological level, by significantly reducing the frequency of bleeding, it preserves joint integrity and minimizes the progression of structural damage. Not only does it imply tangible pain relief, but it also translates into a substantial improvement in the quality of life of individuals, allowing them to participate more actively in various daily activities (Bruyneel, 2023).

Kinesthetic treatment in patients with hemophilia is one of the outstanding examples, where it is described that physiotherapy not only improves joint functionality and reduces pain, but also has a positive impact on the patient's quality of life, allowing greater participation in daily activities (Deniz et al 2022).

Respiratory physiotherapy plays an essential role in the care of patients diagnosed with Duchenne Muscular Dystrophy (DMD), a neuromuscular disease that affects the respiratory muscles, generating significant complications in pulmonary function, the importance in various crucial aspects for the comprehensive care of these patients. It is worth mentioning that DMD leads to progressive respiratory muscle weakness, predisposing to respiratory failure. Respiratory physiotherapy focuses on maintaining lung elasticity and improving respiratory capacity, thus contributing to prevent or delay respiratory failure, one of the main associated complications (Cammarata-Scalisi et al., 2008; Salas, 2014).

Respiratory physiotherapy plays a fundamental preventive role, working on the elimination of bronchial secretions and the performance of specific respiratory exercises. These interventions aim to keep the airways free of obstructions and reduce the incidence of recurrent respiratory infections. An additional benefit lies in improving the function of the accessory muscles of respiration, strengthening these muscles, facilitating more effective breathing, prevention of thoracic deformities to maintain mobility and elasticity of the rib cage, reducing muscle weakness (Demográficas et al., 2023; Jiménez-Jiménez et al., 2015; Lidia & Hernández, 2019; Peron-Magnan, 2023a).

Rehabilitation and intervention in patients with Focal Dystonia represent a comprehensive strategy that goes beyond the mitigation of motor symptoms, offering a series of benefits that positively impact the daily life and quality of life of affected individuals. One of the fundamental aspects addressed is the improvement of motor function. Through adapted exercise and physical therapy programs, affected muscles are strengthened, coordination is improved and greater precision in movements is achieved, allowing more efficient performance of daily tasks.

Another crucial aspect is the reduction of muscle stiffness and tension characteristic of Focal Dystonia. Physiotherapy and specialized interventions employ stretching, myofascial release techniques and manual therapies to relieve tension in muscle tissues, improving flexibility and facilitating greater freedom of movement (Alvarez-Hernandez et al., 2021; Cammarata-Scalisi et al., 2008; Jimenez-Jimenez et al., 2015; Peron-Magnan, 2023b). This approach contributes not only to physical aspects, but also has a positive impact on the patient's overall quality of life. Comprehensive care extends to the emotional and psychological domain, where work is done on the development of coping strategies.

Rehabilitation professionals collaborate with patients to address the emotional challenges associated with Focal Dystonia, fostering resilience and adaptation to the condition. In addition, social participation becomes a goal, because improving functionality and reducing motor symptoms facilitates integration into social and recreational activities, enriching patients' lives, and rehabilitation also plays a crucial role in preventing secondary complications. Early and continuous care contributes to the proper management of Focal Dystonia, reducing the risk of muscle contractures, joint deformities and other health problems that could arise as a consequence of the disease (Jiménez-Jiménez et al., 2015; Peron-

Magnan, 2023b, 2023a; Viteri et al., n/d).

On the other hand, the systematic and structured application of stretching and muscle strengthening techniques is positioned as a comprehensive and highly beneficial strategy to effectively address and improve the symptoms associated with dystonia in musicians. These specialized exercises are precisely designed to specifically target the affected musculature, with the primary goal of enhancing flexibility and strength in specific muscle areas (Cammarata-Scalisi et al., 2008; Peron-Magnan, 2023b).

In the specific context of focal hand dystonia in musicians, the regular incorporation of routines dedicated to stretching and strengthening has shown extremely encouraging results. This therapeutic approach stands out as an effective tool, contributing significantly to the improvement of motor coordination and relief of the involuntary muscle contractions that characterize this condition. The optimization of muscular flexibility and endurance, as the main objective of these practices, not only aims to attenuate symptoms but also seeks to maximize functionality and performance during the execution of musical activities. Among the specific benefits derived from these practices is the reduction of muscle stiffness, which allows for a wider and more fluid range of motion. In addition, improved muscle strength contributes to greater stability and control during musical performance, facilitating the precise execution of fine movements required in instrumental interpretation (Jiménez-Jiménez et al., 2015; Viteri et al., 2020) Likewise, occupational therapy, applied in the context of dystonia, emerges as a comprehensive approach that seeks to provide a variety of benefits both physically and emotionally. It is worth mentioning that, this form of therapy focuses on improving functionality and independence in daily activities of those with dystonia, considering the specific limitations and challenges that this condition may present. From a physical perspective, occupational therapy works on optimizing motor coordination and muscle strength. Professionals in this discipline design personalized interventions that seek to strengthen affected muscles and improve precision in movements, thus contributing to greater dexterity and efficiency in the execution of daily tasks (Peron-Magnan, 2023a; Viteri et al., 2020).

In the psychosocial area, the physiotherapist plays a crucial role in empowering patients, who can continue with prescribed exercises at home, which improves their independence and promotes an integration of rehabilitation into daily life. Learning rehabilitation techniques and participating in their own care generates a sense of control and autonomy, strengthening mental and emotional health. By improving mobility and functionality, social participation is encouraged, reducing the psychosocial impact that hemophilia can have on interpersonal relationships and overall quality of life (Bruyneel, 2023; Peron-Magnan, 2023a).

This psychosocial approach is reflected in every aspect of the physiotherapeutic treatment, showing that the intervention is not limited to physical treatment, but encompasses the patient's entire environment and needs.

Occupational therapy intervention

In the field of physical rehabilitation, occupational therapists design programs tailored to the specific needs of each orphan disease. This may include exercises and techniques that seek to strengthen muscles, improve mobility and prevent the progression of possible physical complications. Through physical and occupational therapies, they seek to maximize the physical functionality of patients, allowing them to perform daily activities with greater independence and autonomy.

With regard to cognitive and sensory development, occupational therapists implement strategies that stimulate and strengthen the mental and sensory abilities of patients with orphan diseases (Menascu et al., 2021; Pallavicini et al., 2018). These approaches include activities designed to improve memory, attention, coordination, and other essential cognitive skills. In addition, sensory techniques are employed to optimize sensory integration and improve the patient's response to environmental stimuli.

It should be noted that the participation and support of family members are fundamental elements in this comprehensive process. Working with family members is fundamental to provide continuous support strategies in the family environment (Lorenzo, 2018; Tejada-Ortigosa et al., 2019), facilitating the implementation of therapeutic recommendations in the patient's daily life. The involvement of family members not only contributes to the success of interventions, but also strengthens the caring and emotionally supportive environment that is essential for the overall well-being of patients with orphan diseases (Lorenzo, 2018).

On the other hand, with respect to the pathophysiological development of orphan diseases, it is essential to highlight the complexity and lack of therapeutic options available to affected patients. The absence of definitive cures and effective palliative treatments, together with the high cost of therapies not covered by national health systems, creates a challenging situation that often leads to the social and institutional abandonment of these patients (Bravo et al., 2014; Lorenzo, 2018; Torriente et al., 2021; Waldo et al., 2021).

Despite these challenges, it is important to recognize the significant role that occupational therapy plays in maintaining and improving the quality of life of people affected by orphan diseases. These have become a key element in addressing the specific needs of these patients, providing personalized interventions that contribute to mitigating the negative impacts of the disease.

In contrast to the lack of definitive medical solutions, occupational therapy offers a holistic approach that considers both physical as well as emotional and cognitive dimensions of health. These therapies seek to optimize patients' daily functionality, promote independence in daily activities and improve their psychosocial well-being (Lorenzo, 2018; Rivera & Vaquero, 2022).

Mobilization and physical therapy are key aspects that are part of care and implementation of early mobilization techniques helps prevent muscle atrophy and contributes to the maintenance of joint mobility. Nurses work closely with physiotherapists to adapt mobilization plans according to the patient's progression, seeking to preserve physical functionality (Rodriguez 2019).

Moreover, within the framework of comprehensive care for patients with orphan diseases, the intervention of occupational therapists plays an indispensable role in addressing various dimensions of the health and well-being of affected individuals. These professional occupational therapy experts apply personalized strategies to improve patients' quality of life, focusing on physical rehabilitation and cognitive and sensory development. In addition, occupational therapy addresses the emotional and psychological needs of individuals with dystonia. Adjusting to a chronic condition can create challenges to emotional well-being, and occupational therapists work collaboratively with patients to develop effective coping strategies. This not only helps reduce negative emotional impact, such as anxiety or frustration, but also promotes resilience and positive adjustment to the condition. Another fundamental aspect of occupational therapy is its focus on improving overall quality of life. Occupational therapists work on adapting environments and routines to facilitate participation in daily life. This may include recommendations for home adjustments, modifications in the way certain activities are performed, and the introduction of tools or technologies that facilitate autonomy and social inclusion (Tejada- Ortigosa et al., 2019).

Speech Therapy Intervention

Children with orphan diseases often present with speech and language disorders that can vary in severity and manifestation. These disorders are frequently related to specific genetic mutations that affect both language development and other cognitive aspects. Early identification and accurate characterization of these disorders are crucial to implement effective therapeutic interventions and improve the quality of life of children with an orphan disease.

Speech therapy in children with orphan diseases is an area of research that seeks to improve communication skills in children with rare and complex conditions. The following are key findings from several studies on this topic taking into account their clinical characteristics, for example, regarding the efficacy of Intensive Interventions: both the Nuffield Dyspraxia Program-3 (NDP-3) and Rapid Syllable Transitions Treatment (ReST) showed improvements in word accuracy in children with childhood apraxia of speech when administered intensively (Mongan, Murray, & Liégeois, 2018). Regarding Speech and Language Therapy in Cerebral Palsy: Speech and language therapies can improve communication skills in children with cerebral palsy, although evidence is limited and more studies are needed to confirm their effectiveness (Pennington, Goldbart, Marshall, 2004). Another aspect such as therapy for Childhood Dysarthria: We found no randomized controlled trials demonstrating the effectiveness of speech and language therapy interventions in improving speech intelligibility in children with dysarthria acquired before the age of three (Pennington, Parker, et al., 2016), as they relate to interventions for Primary Speech and Language Disorders: Speech and language therapy is effective for children with phonological and expressive vocabulary difficulties, but the evidence is less clear for receptive syntax difficulties (Law, Garrett, Nye, 2003), along these same lines therapy for Children with Cleft Lip and/or Palate: Speech and language therapy can improve speech production in children with cleft lip and cleft palate, although the evidence is variable and more studies are needed (Sand, Hagberg, Lohmander, 2022), however, it was found that in some occasions it improves markedly according to its frequency, finally the Online Speech Therapy systems (Teletherapy): The option of receiving online therapy or teletherapy can be beneficial for children with communication disorders as a consequence of an orphan disease, especially in settings where there is a shortage of speech therapists.(Attwell, Bennin, Tekinerdogan, 2022).

From the above, it is concluded that speech therapy may be beneficial for children with various orphan diseases, although the evidence varies depending on the specific condition and type of intervention. Intensive and proactive therapies show further progress and hope in the midst of the struggle to improve each of the specific conditions, but more rigorous studies are needed to confirm their effectiveness and determine best practices.

Nursing Intervention

On the other hand, nursing care is a fundamental pillar in the comprehensive approach and long-term improvement of bronchopulmonary dysplasia (Lidia & Hernández, 2019) in neonates, especially in those born prematurely. Continuous monitoring, by constantly assessing vital parameters such as respiratory rate and oxygen saturation, provides the ability to detect any signs of respiratory deterioration in its early stages, allowing timely and effective interventions. Respiratory support, which involves the precise administration of oxygen and careful management of ventilation, stands as a crucial component to maintain adequate saturation levels and favor optimal lung function, thus contributing to respiratory stability in neonates affected by BPD (Lidia & Hernández, 2019). In addition, nursing care extends beyond the neonate, encompassing a crucial component of emotional support for parents. Providing clear and understandable information about the infant's condition, along with encouraging parental involvement in daily care, strengthens family adjustment and contributes to overall emotional well-being.

Nutrition Intervention

Nutrition is fundamental in the maintenance of human health and well-being. Its importance is magnified when considering its direct link to the prevention and management of various diseases, including rare diseases. Rare diseases, characterized by their low prevalence and often clinical complexity, present unique challenges for patients and healthcare professionals. In this context, nutrition becomes an essential component in improving the quality of life of those affected by these diseases.

In the nutritional area, specific care seeks to overcome the difficulties associated with respiratory fatigue, implementing strategies such as the administration of food in smaller and more frequent portions. In more complex cases, enteral nutrition is used to ensure that neonates receive the nutrients necessary for their development. Respiratory physiotherapy plays a crucial role by incorporating techniques such as percussion and vibration, which not only improve lung expansion, but also prevent complications related to the accumulation of secretions, thus favoring more efficient breathing (Rosa Güell et al., 2007).

Infection prevention, through rigorous control measures, is essential to protect these neonates, who, due to their condition, are more susceptible to respiratory infections. The strategies implemented seek to safeguard their well-being and prevent further complications. Early stimulation and development-centered care translate into significant benefits, promoting skin-to-skin contact and creating environments that favor sensory development, contributing positively to cardiovascular and respiratory stability (Rosa Güell et al., 2007).

It should also be emphasized that good nutrition and the support of family members play a key role in the development of the well-being of people affected by Crohn's disease. A balanced diet adapted to the specific needs of this inflammatory bowel condition contributes to maintaining health and managing symptoms. The presence of committed family members facilitates the implementation of proper eating habits, offering essential emotional support, creating an environment of understanding and collaboration, helping to mitigate the psychological and emotional impact of the disease (Lorenzo, 2018; Tejada-Ortigosa et al., 2019).

Home or domiciliary intervention

Likewise, the implementation of therapies at home has become a crucial component for the improvement of muscles and movement in people with systemic impairments. This therapeutic approach, combined with rehabilitation in physiotherapeutic centers (Fernandez & Arcos, 2019; Menascu et al., 2021; Peron-Magnan, 2023), creates a comprehensive program that addresses the specific needs of each individual. In physiotherapy centers, professionals design personalized treatment plans based on a thorough assessment of the patient's abilities and limitations. These include exercises focused on strengthening specific muscle groups, improving joint mobility and enhancing compromised motor skills. Physiotherapists use advanced techniques and specialized equipment to optimize rehabilitation outcomes (Mamaladze et al., 2022; Menascu et al., 2021).

In the home setting, exercises prescribed during in-center therapies become daily tasks that the patient performs at home. These exercises are selected to address specific areas of functional weakness or limitation, and are adapted according to individual progress (Hermoso, 2021). Consistency in performing these exercises contributes significantly to muscle strengthening and improvement of motor skills over time. The benefits of combining rehabilitation in physiotherapeutic centers with therapies at home are diverse (Antonia & Nadal, 2018; Hermoso, 2021). Since they guarantee the correct and proper application of the technique, the safe progression of the exercises. In addition, the home environment offers the opportunity to practice the skills learned in everyday situations, promoting a greater transfer of these skills (Peron-Magnan, 2023a; Scaturro et al., 2021).

The flexibility and adaptability of home therapies are also key aspects. Patients can incorporate rehabilitation sessions into their daily routines, which facilitates the integration of rehabilitation into their lifestyle. This not only improves adherence to treatment, but also fosters greater autonomy and empowerment for the patient in their recovery process. On the other hand, the implementation of home therapies has become a crucial component for the improvement of muscle and movement in people with systemic impairments. This therapeutic approach, combined with rehabilitation in physical therapy centers, creates a comprehensive program that addresses the specific needs of each individual (Cason, 2012; Forsyth et al., 2020; López-Casaus et al., 2021; Torriente et al., 2021). These plans usually include a variety of exercises focused on strengthening specific muscle groups, improving joint mobility and enhancing compromised motor skills. Physical therapists use advanced techniques and specialized equipment to optimize rehabilitation outcomes (Alvarez-Hernandez et al., 2021; Deniz et al., 2022; Hermans & Dolan, 2020).

The benefits of combining rehabilitation in physiotherapy centers with therapies at home are diverse. Constant supervision by physical therapists in the centers ensures proper correction of technique and safe progression of exercises (Alvarez-Hernandez et al., 2021; Deniz et al., 2022). In addition, the home setting offers the opportunity to practice the skills learned in everyday situations, promoting a greater transfer of these skills to the patient's day-to-day life. The flexibility and adaptability of home therapies are also key aspects. Patients can incorporate rehabilitation sessions into their daily routines, which facilitates the integration of rehabilitation into their lifestyle. This not only improves adherence to treatment, but also fosters greater autonomy and empowerment for the patient in their recovery process (Deniz et al., 2022).

Social Work Intervention

One of the highlights is the emotional support that Social Work provides to both patients and their families. ALS can generate significant emotional stresses, and the social worker becomes a key resource to help people cope with these challenges, offering guidance and support in difficult times, in addition, Social Work intervention strengthens the role of the family in the rehabilitation process. It provides tools and strategies to cope with changes in family dynamics, fosters effective communication and promotes resilience in the family environment (Pallavicini et al., 2018).

On the other hand, Social Work intervention in the rehabilitation process of individuals affected by ALS plays an essential role in addressing not only the medical aspects, but also the complex emotional and social dimensions of the disease. The benefits of having Social Work professionals are diverse and range from facilitating access to practical resources and services to providing comprehensive emotional support. Professional care assessment is conducted in a comprehensive manner, considering the physical and psychosocial needs of each patient. Close collaboration with other health professionals ensures coordinated and tailored care, contributing to the overall well-being of the individual (Waldo et al., 2021).

Intervention by medical specialties

Likewise, the management of pediatric patients diagnosed with microtia in the Otolaryngology service is characterized by a comprehensive approach that thoroughly addresses every aspect of the condition. The complete evaluation of each patient goes beyond the identification of microtia, considering the possible implications for hearing and other functions related to aural anatomy. This comprehensive approach allows for accurate diagnosis and the formulation of highly personalized treatment plans tailored to the specific conditions of each child. Pediatric care in this context is distinguished by a unique sensitivity to the emotional and psychological needs of both children and their families (Guillen de la Colina, 2018). Management of microtia involves effective communication with parents, providing them with clear information and setting realistic expectations about procedures and treatments. This collaborative approach facilitates understanding and family involvement in the care process.

The advantage of having a multidisciplinary team is essential in the management of microtia in children. Close collaboration between otolaryngologists, plastic surgeons, audiologists and other specialists allows for a comprehensive approach to the various dimensions of the condition. From aesthetics to hearing function, this holistic approach optimizes outcomes and ensures comprehensive and coordinated care. The Otolaryngology service stands out not only for its advanced clinical approach, but also for the incorporation of cutting-edge technologies that support the most current procedures and treatments for microtia. Innovative surgical techniques, such as auricular reconstruction, are an integral part of the treatment offerings, seeking to improve both the aesthetic appearance and hearing function of patients (Demográficas et al., 2023).

Patient-centered care is a hallmark feature that permeates the entire process of microtia management in the pediatric ENT service (Guillen, 2018). The medical and nursing staff strives to create a comfortable and friendly environment specifically designed for children, thus helping to reduce the anxiety and stress associated with medical procedures. This comprehensive care not only addresses patients' immediate needs, but also lays the foundation for sustained improvements in their long-term health and quality of life (Demographics et al., 2023; Guillen, 2018).

Other special conditions such as fibromyalgia

With respect to fibromyalgia, a disease of unknown origin, which significantly impacts the quality of life of those who suffer from it, has led to the development of therapeutic interventions that are deployed in various areas to address symptoms and improve functionality in different aspects of daily life. Occupational therapy in fibromyalgia patients plays a central role in the care of people with fibromyalgia, focusing on strategies that support occupational performance, promote personal autonomy and improve quality of life. This approach involves working on meaningful activities for each individual, adapting environments and routines to optimize functionality in daily and work activities (Vila Paz et al., 2021).

Sleep management emerges as a key piece in the approach to fibromyalgia. Strategies such as sleep hygiene, relaxation techniques and cognitive-behavioral therapies are implemented to improve sleep quality, reduce fatigue and mitigate other associated symptoms, becoming an essential component of this intervention. In addition, recreational therapy is incorporated to promote leisure activities adapted to individual abilities and needs, providing not only distraction and pleasure, but also contributing to stress reduction and mood improvement, crucial aspects in the management of fibromyalgia (Vila Paz et al., 2021).

Given the characteristics of this disease to generate social isolation, psychosocial interventions focus on strengthening communication skills, setting boundaries and managing stress in social contexts. Support groups and patient networks offer a valuable space to share experiences and receive emotional support (Pallavicini et al., 2018). In addition to psychosocial interventions, pharmacological treatments are used to manage symptoms such as pain and fatigue. Combining pharmacological treatments with non-pharmacological approaches, such as physiotherapy and adaptive exercises, proves beneficial in improving physical functionality and managing pain in the context of fibromyalgia (Vila Paz et al., 2021).

Intervention focused on needs

Another key element is care focused on the specific needs of each patient. Nurses tailor care according to the variability in the clinical presentation of GBS (Carrasco & Fernanda, 2020; Rodriguez, 2019), responding in an individualized manner to each patient's unique challenges and symptoms. This personalization contributes to more effective management and a more positive care experience. Emotional support is a hallmark feature of nursing care for patients with OS (Fernandez & Arcos, 2019). They play an essential role in providing emotional support, explaining the course of the disease, and fostering effective communication between the patient and the medical team (Huasasasquiche et al., 2017; Mamaladze et al., 2022).

CONCLUSIONS

The biopsychosocial theories and models present in the analyzed paper offer important contributions to the field of rehabilitation and intervention in orphan diseases. Authors such as Flores highlight the relevance of implementing comprehensive neuropsychological rehabilitation programs to mitigate the cognitive sequelae derived from diseases such as ischemic cerebrovascular disease in middle-aged adults. This prospective and quantitative approach demonstrated significant improvements in several cognitive and emotional areas, highlighting the efficacy of interventions based on biopsychosocial models.

In addition, the systematic review carried out with methodological rigor, following the guidelines of Reporting Items for Systematic Reviews and Meta-Analyses (PRISMA), ensures the validity and reliability of the results obtained. This structured methodology not only facilitates the collection of high quality information, but also enables an accurate and complete synthesis of advances in rehabilitation, intervention and biopsychosocial models related to orphan diseases. Furthermore, the diversity of the scientific literature used in the review contributes to a solid foundation for the conclusions and provides a comprehensive and contextualized view of the interactions between rare diseases and rehabilitation. By considering multiple perspectives and approaches, the overall understanding of orphan diseases is enriched and a more holistic approach to patient care is promoted.

In the detailed exploration of this article, an exhaustive analysis of the fundamental processes related to rehabilitation and intervention in the context of orphan diseases has been carried out. In addition, the application of the biopsychosocial model has been addressed to comprehensively understand the complexity that these conditions present in the lives of those who suffer from them. This holistic approach not only sheds light on the medical aspects of these diseases, but also highlights the importance of considering the psychological and social aspects in the design of effective treatment strategies.

In the course of research, several orphan diseases have been identified and explored in depth, including multiple sclerosis, Guillain-Barré syndrome and psoriatic rheumatism. Delving into the specific characteristics of each of these conditions not only enriches our understanding of their pathophysiology, but also allows for a better appreciation of the individual needs of patients. This detailed knowledge serves as a cornerstone for the design of personalized interventions and the implementation of treatments that are precisely tailored to the particularities of each case.

By broadening the view on orphan diseases, this article contributes significantly to the scientific field and to the development of essential information for the design of more effective therapeutic strategies. The information gathered becomes a valuable resource for healthcare professionals, researchers, and those involved in healthcare decision making. By thoroughly understanding the complexities of these diseases, the way is paved for the creation of more effective and personalized treatment protocols, thus improving the quality of life for those facing these challenging medical conditions.

REFERENCES

Álvarez-Hernández, D. A., García-Rodríguez-Arana, R., Ortiz-Hernández, A., Álvarez- Sánchez, M., Wu, M., Mejia, R., Martínez-Juárez, L. A., Montoya, A., Gallardo- Rincon, H., Vázquez-López, R., & Fernández-Presas, A. M. (2021). A systematic review of historical and current trends in Chagas disease. In Therapeutic Advances in Infectious Disease (Vol. 8). SAGE Publications Ltd. https://doi.org/10.1177/20499361211033715

Antonia, M., & Nadal, P. (2018). The resources of the CCEE Pinyol Vermell (ASPACE) for the improvement of communication of students with Infantile Cerebral Palsy or Rare Diseases. Final degree work. Universitat de les Illes Balears.

Bove, R. M., Rush, G., Zhao, C., Rowles, W., Garcha, P., Morrissey, J., ... & Anguera, J. (2019). A videogame-based digital therapeutic to improve processing speed in people with multiple sclerosis: a feasibility study. *Neurology and therapy, 8,* 135145. https://doi.org/10.6084/m9.figshare.7363955.

Bravo, J., Chávez, V., Cid, D., Montecino, R., Toro, X., & Sepúlveda, R. (2014). Occupational therapy in labor inclusion: Experiences at the local level. Revista Chilena de Terapia Ocupacional, 14(1), 111. https://doi.org/10.5354/0719-5346.2014.32396

Bruyneel, A.V. (2023). Assessment of proprioception: tests of statesthesia and kinesthesia in clinical practice. EMC - Kinesitherapy - Physical Medicine, 44(1), 115. https://doi.org/10.1016/s1293-2965(22)47314-2.

Cammarata-Scalisi, F., Camacho, N., Alvarado, J., & Lacruz-Rengel, M. A. (2008). Duchenne muscular dystrophy, clinical presentation. Revista Chilena de Pediatria, 79(5), 495-501. https://doi.org/10.4067/S0370-41062008000500007.

Carrasco, M., & Fernanda, M. (2020). Orphaned Diseases Orphaned Diseases. https://doi. org/10.5281/zenodo.4263347.

Cason, J. (2012). Telehealth opportunities in occupational therapy through the affordable care act. American Journal of Occupational Therapy, 66(2), 131-136. https://doi.org/10.5014/AJOT.2012.662001

Castañeda Guillot, C. (2023). Rare diseases in childhood. Gastroenterological view. Revista Cubana de Pediatría, 95. https://orcid.org/0000-0001- 0925-5211.

Deniz, V., Guzel, N. A., Lobet, S., Antmen, A. B., Sasmaz, H. I., Kilci, A., Boyraz, O. C., Gunasli, O., & Kurdak, S. S. (2022). Effects of a supervised therapeutic exercise program on musculoskeletal health and gait in patients with haemophilia: A pilot study. Haemophilia, 28(1), 166-175. https://doi.org/10.1111/HAE. 14444

Farrús, M. (2023). Automatic Speech Recognition in L2 Learning: A Review Based on PRISMA Methodology. Languages, 8(4), 242. https://doi.org/10.3390/languages8040242

Fernández, M. J. N., & Arcos, D. P. R. (2019). Video games with a binocular approach: a new trend for amblyopia treatment. *Science and Technology for Eye and Vision Health, 17(1),* 5. https://doi.org/10.19052/sv.vol17.issL6

Forsyth, A., Blamey, G., Lobet, S., & McLaughlin, P. (2020). Practical Guidance for Non-Specialist Physical Therapists Managing People with Hemophilia and Musculoskeletal Complications. Health, 12(02), 158-179. https://doi.org/10.4236/health.2020.122014

Guillen de la Colina, R. D. (2018). Correlation of microtia and the degree of hypoacusis in pediatric and adolescent patient. Degree work specialty of oral and maxillofacial surgery. Autonomous University of Nuevo Leon.

Hermans, C., & Dolan, G. (2020). Pharmacokinetics in routine haemophilia clinical practice: rationale and modalities-a practical review. Therapeutic Advances in

Hematology, 11. https://doi.org/10.1177/2040620720966888

Huasasquiche, M., Alonso, D., Morales Martínez, L., & Engels, M. (2017). CERVICAL DYSTONIA: PHYSIOTHERAPY TREATMENT Research work Professional Sufficiency Work To opt for the Professional Degree. Inv. D-398 MFN 7614 thesis.

Hermoso, Á. L. (2021). European regulations on orphan drugs.

Hirmas Adauy, M., Poffald Angulo, L., Jasmen Sepúlveda, A. M., Aguilera Sanhueza, X., Delgado Becerra, I., & Vega Morales, J. (2013). Barriers and facilitators of access to health care: a qualitative systematic review. Pan American Journal of Public Health, 33, 223-229.

Jiménez-Jiménez, F. J., Alonso-Navarro, H., Piudo, M. R. L., & Hernández, J. A. B. (2015). Movement disorders (III): Chorea syndromes and dystonia. Medicine (Spain), 11(74), 4439-4453. https://doi.org/10.1016/bmed.2015.02.012.

Kalb, R., Brown, T. R., Coote, S., Costello, K., Dalgas, U., Garmon, E., Giesser, B., Halper, J., Karpatkin, H., Keller, J., Ng, A. V., Pilutti, L. A., Rohrig, A., Van Asch, P., Zackowski, K., & Motl, R. W. (2020). Exercise and lifestyle physical activity recommendations for people with multiple sclerosis throughout the disease course. Multiple Sclerosis Journal, 26(12), 1459-1469. https://doi.org/10.1177/1352458520915629

Lidia, C., & Hernández, M. (2019). Effectiveness of the educational program on prevention and control of nosocomial infections in knowledge and practices for nurses of the neonatal intensive care unit of the Sergio Bernales Comas National Hospital July 2014 - July 2015. National University Hermilio Valdizán. http://repositorio.unheval.edu.pe/handle/20.500.13080/4412

Llanos, C., Pardo, J., & Romero, O. M. (2020). Challenges for the social inclusion of patients with orphan diseases. Monografia como opción de grado. Psychology Program. National Open and Distance University UNAD

López-Casaus, A., Jiménez-Sánchez, C., Esteban-Repiso, L., Lafuente-Ureta, R.,

Cordova-Alegre, P., & Alfaro-Gervon, F. (2021). Hemophilia patient experience in a physical therapy-guided health education intervention: A mixed-method design. Healthcare (Switzerland), 9(12). https://doi.org/10.3390/healthcare9121728. https://doi.org/10.3390/healthcare9121728.

Lorenzo Barbeito, L. (2018). Occupational therapy and family-centered practice: occupational changes and priorities of families of children with rare diseases. http s://ruc.udc.es/dspace/handle/2183/20836

Mamaladze, T., (2022). Neuropsychological assessment and rehabilitation in multiple sclerosis. Final Master's thesis in Neuropsychology. Open University of Catalonia. https://openaccess.uoc.edu/bitstream/10609/146646/2/tamamaladzeTFM0622memoria. pdf

María, A., & Chiriboga, D. (n/d). UNIVERSIDAD SAN FRANCISCO DE QUITO USFQ College of Health Sciences CURRICULAR INTEGRATION WORK GRADING SHEET Development of cases of community nutrition, life cycle, Crohn's disease and Down Syndrome. http://bit.ly/COPETheses.

Mejia, C. R., Valladares-Garrido, M. J., Valladares-Garrido, D., & Bazán-Ruiz, S. (2018). Response to the possible identification bias of patients with rare or high-cost diseases. Salud Uninorte, 34(1), 248-250. https://doi.org/10.14482/sun.34.Ln 205

Menascu, S., Aloni, R., Dolev, M., Magalashvili, D., Gutman, K., Dreyer-Alster, S., Tarpin-Bernard, F., Achiron, R., Harari, G., & Achiron, A. (2021). Targeted cognitive game training enhances cognitive performance in multiple sclerosis patients treated with interferon beta 1-a. Journal of NeuroEngineering and Rehabilitation, 18(1). https://doi.org/10.1186/s12984-021-00968-3. https://doi.org/10.1186/s12984-021-00968-3.

Pallavicini, F., Ferrari, A., & Mantovani, F. (2018). Video games for well-being: A systematic review on the application of computer games for cognitive and emotional training in the adult population. In Frontiers in Psychology (Vol. 9, NOV Issue). Frontiers Media S.A. https://doi.org/10.3389/fpsyg.2018.02127.

Peron-Magnan, T. (2023). Rehabilitation of dystonia. EMC - Kinesitherapy - Physical Medicine, 44(2), 1-15. https://doi.org/10.1016/S1293-2965(23)47624-4.

Pizarro Laborda, P., Santana López, A., & Vial Lavín, B. (2013). Family participation and its linkage in the learning processes of children in school contexts. *Diversitas: perspectives in psychology, 9*(2), 271-287.

Posada, M., Martin-Arribas, C., Ramírez, A., Villaverde, A., & Abaitua, I. (2008). Rare diseases: Concept, epidemiology and current situation in Spain. In *Anales del sistema sanitario de Navarra* (Vol. 31, pp. 9-20). Government of Navarra. Department of Health. https://doi.org/10.1111/hae.13393

Camelo, L. R., Carpio, M. T., Camelo, L. R., & Carpio, M. T. (2023) Systematic Review of the Effectiveness of Physical Therapy Intervention through Telerehabilitation in Users with Neuromuscular System Impairment. Degree work for physiotherapy degree. University of Santander

Rivera, S. B., & Vaquero, M. T. (2022). Occupational therapy process in the follow-up of high-risk premature infants following NICU admission in the province of Santa Fe. https://rid.ugr.edu.ar/handle/20.500.14125/493

Rodriguez, B. (2019). Nursing staff performance in patients with rare diseases. Undergraduate thesis. Nursing program. University of Valladolid. https://uvadoc.uva.es/handle/10324/36797

Rosa Güell, M., Avendano, M., Fraser, J., & Goldstein, R. (2007). Pulmonary and nonpulmonary alterations in Duchenne muscular dystrophy. Archives of Bronchopneumology, 43(10), 557-561. https://doi.org/10.1157/13110881.

Salas, A. C. (2014). Duchenne muscular dystrophy. Anales de Pediatria Continuada, 12(2), 47-54. https://doi.org/10.1016/S1696-2818(14)70168-4.

Sampieri, H., Fernández Collado, R., & Baptista Lucio, C. (2004). Research Methodology.

Scaturro, D., Benedetti, M. G., Lomonaco, G., Tomasello, S., Giuseppina Farella, M. G., Frizziero, A., & Mauro, G. L. (2021). Effectiveness of rehabilitation on pain and function in people affected by hemophilia. Medicine (United States), 100(50), E27863. https://doi.org/10.1097/MD.0000000000027863

Tejada-Ortigosa, E. M., Flores-Rojas, K., Moreno-Quintana, L., Muñoz-Villanueva, M. C., Pérez-Navero, J. L., & Gil-Campos, M. (2019). Health and socio-educational needs of the families and children with rare metabolic diseases: Qualitative study in a tertiary hospital. Anales de Pediatria, 90(1), 42-50. https://doi.org/10.1016/j.anpedi.2018.03.003

Torriente Herrera, N., Marianne Sánchez Savigñón, I. I., & María Franco, A. I. (2021). Dystonia and occupational therapeutic care Dystonia and occupational therapeutic.

Vila Paz, A., Sergio, E. D., Santos, D., & Riego, C. E. U. (2021). Impact of biopsychosocial factors on the quality of life of people diagnosed with fibromyalgia. https://ruc.udc.es/dspace/handle/2183/29514

Viteri, J., Morales Carrasco, A., Jácome, M., Vaca, G., Tubón, I., Rodríguez, V., ... & Vinueza, D. (2020). Orphan diseases. Archivos Venezolanos de Farmacología y Terapéutica, 39(5), 627-634. https://doi. org/10.5281/zenodo.4263347

Waldo, T. O., San, E., & Bravo, J. (2021). Systematization of Occupational Therapy interventions in Telehealth modality during pandemic. An experience of the Social and Labor Inclusion Program at the Friends of Jesus Foundation. Contexto, 7(7), 13-30. https://doi.org/10.5281/ZENODO.5711698

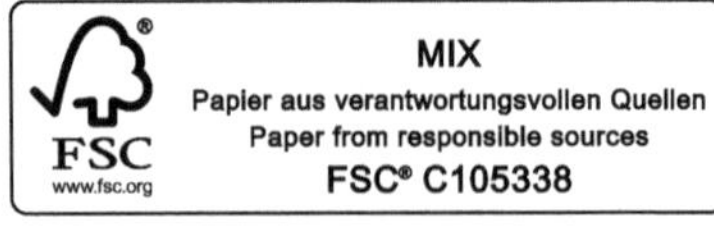

Printed by Books on Demand GmbH, Norderstedt / Germany